Facts About

Breast Cancer

Written and edited by
Dr Robert Leonard
Consultant in Clinical Oncology
Western General Hospital, Edinburgh, UK
with
Fatima Patel,
Mediscript Ltd.

In memory of Shushi and Lena.

The views and opinions in this book are based on current knowledge and do not necessarily reflect the views of the publishers or any other manufacturer of pharmaceutical products mentioned herein.

Key Facts about Breast Cancer
is published by
Mediscript
1 Mountview Court
310 Friern Barnet Lane
London N20 0LD
UK

ISBN 1-871211-51-4

Contents

1 *Introduction*

Breast cancer is a disease of the cells in the breast tissue and is a common illness that can affect all age groups of the adult female population. This book aims to explain, in simple terms, the key facts about breast cancer to aid understanding of this widespread disease. It will cover important facts, such as how cancer develops and how this relates specifically to breast cancer. It will give the current facts and figures of how many women are affected or likely to be affected, at what age and due to what risk factors. It will also cover the processes involved in screening, diagnosis, prognosis and treatment, together with information relating to the wide network of support groups.

The main aim of this book is to provide an enlightened view of breast cancer based on the latest research data and to help patients and their families to cope as best as possible with the condition.

The book will provide a clear understanding of breast cancer in a form that can be read at home in your own time. Although you may be told most of what is contained here by your doctors or nurses, this book will help to consolidate the discussion you will have with your medical team and guide you towards asking them the appropriate questions.

Various medical terms are explained fully in the text and there is also a comprehensive glossary of terms provided at the end of the book.

2 *What is cancer?*

We are all familiar with the word 'cancer' and to most of us it is associated with a certain aura of a serious illness, usually terminating in death. How true this impression is has to be weighed against current statistics: although around 300 000 patients are diagnosed as having cancer each year in the United Kingdom, the death rate from cancer is around 164 000 per year (just above 50% of all those diagnosed with cancer in the United Kingdom) and may be falling.

Few of us would be able to provide an accurate definition of cancer. In Latin 'cancer' means a crab, and it was originally used to describe a creeping ulcer that spreads gradually, eating away and destroying body tissues in its path. In actual fact, cancer develops as a result of an abnormal cell, which multiplies to produce millions of cells to form a lump or tumour.

Several other words — tumour, neoplasm and malignant growth – are sometimes used to try to avoid the use of the emotive word 'cancer'. To use the word tumour as a substitute for cancer is not strictly accurate as the word tumour means simply a 'swelling'. A tumour may or may not be malignant, that is it may or may not be cancerous. So, to be more accurate, 'malignant tumour' or 'malignant growth' describes a cancer and 'benign tumour' or 'benign growth' describes a relatively harmless swelling.

A benign tumour is one that does not spread into surrounding areas of the body or to other parts of the body whereas a malignant tumour or cancer can spread from its original site into the surrounding tissues and to other parts of the body. However, some malignant disorders, such as leukaemia — a form of blood cancer — never form a tumour or swelling. The word neoplasm, derived from Greek, means 'new growth'. In discussions about cancer you may also hear the words 'carcinoma' and 'sarcoma'. These are medical terms for certain cancers that form in a particular way or in specific parts of the body.

The important characteristics of malignant disorders, that is of cancers, as opposed to benign growths, are:

1 **Cancers are genetic disorders**

A cancer arises from a normal cell when something happens to the genetic material of the cell in the nucleus, ie in the deoxy-ribonucleic acid or DNA. Genes are the elements of DNA that determine an individual's characteristics, from eye colour to height and, possibly, the tendency to develop particular diseases, including cancer. The abnormal DNA or gene sends a signal to instruct the cell to divide and to ignore any controlling signals from surrounding cells or hormones.

What precisely triggers this change is largely unknown, but abnormal genes are being revealed in an increasing number of cancers and their functions are now being understood. This is likely to be crucially important for developing new screening techniques and even treatment plans for the future.

2 Continuous growth in the tissues or flesh surrounding the tumour

This growth at the site of origin of the tumour may produce some of the following symptoms:

- Local swelling (common).
- Pain (sometimes).
- Other complications, such as bleeding, due to spread of the growth into blood vessels (common in lung cancers).
- Obstruction (for example, blockage of the bowel due to bowel cancer).

3 The tendency to spread to distant sites of the body to produce secondary tumours (called metastases)

This occurs when cancers invade blood vessels or lymph channels at the site of their original growth and get carried to other sites of the body in these transport systems. The lymphatic system consists of a network of lymph glands, also known as lymph nodes, which are connected by minute lymph vessels. This system is vitally concerned with fighting infection and disease in all areas of the body. Lymph glands are situated all over the body, including the armpits and groin. The most commonly recognised lymph glands are the tonsils.

4 The likelihood that, without effective treatment, the cancer will shorten the patient's life

Effective treatment can mean surgery, radiotherapy, chemotherapy or any combination of these. Whether or not other 'typical' symptoms of cancer, such as loss of weight and loss of energy or appetite, occur is very variable between cancers and between different patients. These symptoms are not seen in early breast cancer.

The diagnosis of malignancy, however, can be made while the condition is still treatable and curable, before it has spread to distant sites. This diagnosis of malignancy at the 'primary' site is dependent upon the expertise of the pathologist (a specialist in examining cells and tissues under a microscope), whose input into the initial management, although unseen by the patient, is critically important. This is the reason for obtaining a small piece of tissue by performing a tissue biopsy (see Section 4.2); a scan or x-ray will not suffice.

3 *Breast cancer*

3.1 What is breast cancer?

The breasts are normally made up of fat and gland tissue divided into lobes (see Figure 1). These lobes contain milk ducts that terminate in the nipple. The breasts are attached to the muscles of the chest by fine ligaments. Each breast is also supplied with blood through a network of arteries. The breast tissue extends to the armpits, which contain a collection of lymph glands (see Figure 2).

All glandular tissue in the breast is made up of individual cells, which normally grow and reproduce in the breast under the control of hormones. Sometimes this process gets out of control and an abnormal cell develops. The cell continues to reproduce and builds up into a lump or swelling. This is a tumour.

Tumours or lumps in the breasts can be either benign or malignant and most breast lumps are benign tumours. Malignant tumours in the breast — breast cancers — tend to start in the cells that make up the milk ducts.

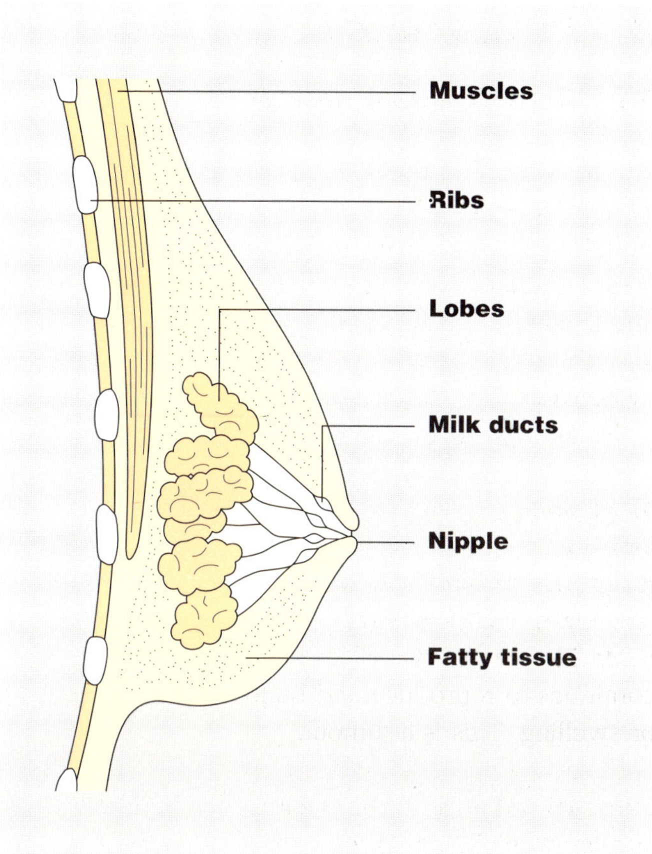

Figure 1. Breasts comprise fat and gland tissue

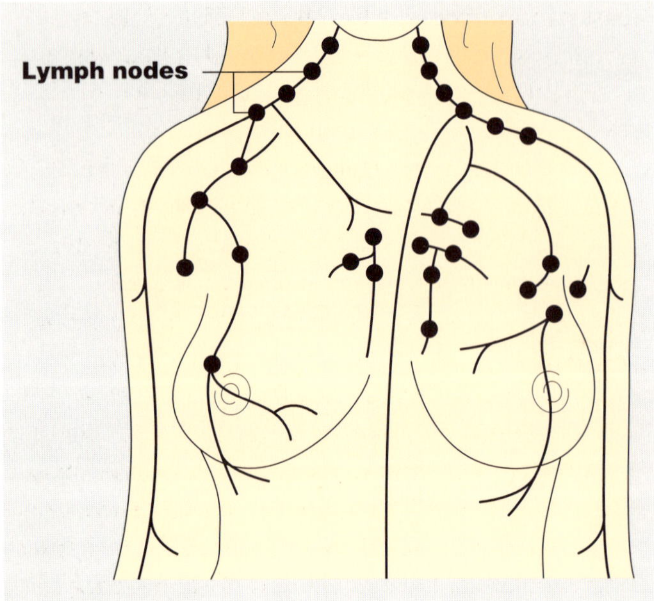

Figure 2. Distribution of lymph nodes in the upper body

3.2 How common is breast cancer?

Breast cancer is common. About one woman in 12 in the United Kingdom will contract breast cancer in her lifetime and it therefore constitutes a major health problem, with around 25 000 new cases per year in Britain and around 15 000 deaths. The overall incidence of breast cancer appears to be rising, with a recorded 11% increase in the years 1968–1978 and with further increases since then.

Breast cancer accounts for around 25% of all cancers in women and for 20% of all cancer deaths; it is the most common cause of death in women between the ages of 44 and 50 in the United Kingdom. Indeed, the United Kingdom has the highest death rates from breast cancer in the world, with deaths in England and Wales slightly greater than in Scotland. Incidence rates vary widely throughout the world, with very high incidences in North America and Northern Europe and low incidences in Asia and parts of Africa. It seems likely that these differences are more due to diet and cultural or geographical differences rather than racial characteristics. Japanese or Hawaiian women who settle in the United States have daughters and granddaughters whose likelihood of developing breast cancer follows the United States pattern, despite not intermarrying.

Nonetheless, the incidence of breast cancer has to be set in the context of benign breast disease associated with lumps. Nine out of ten women who go to their doctor with breast lumps have a benign disorder, not cancer. Furthermore, normal changes associated with the menstrual cycle can make breasts feel lumpy and it is for this reason that breast examination (see Section 4.4) should be done a few days after a menstrual period. Any new lumps or changes should be investigated.

3.3 Age of onset

The risk of developing breast cancer is very rare in women in their 20s, rare in those in their 30s and becomes increasingly common thereafter. It can be said to occur at any time between the ages of 30 and 90 years. The relative risk doubles between the ages of 45 and 75 years. There is a slight flattening of the risk around the menopausal age, but thereafter it increases steadily into old age. It is twice as common in patients in their 70s compared with those in their 40s.

3.4 Risks and causes

A number of specific life events have been associated with an enhanced risk of breast cancer and these are listed below:

1 **The length of the fertile period (ie from first period until menopause)**
A woman who has her menopause at the age of 55 years has twice the risk of developing breast cancer than a woman whose menopause was at the age of 45 years.

2 **Age at first completed pregnancy**
This is also important, with younger age being somewhat protective and older age (first child

after age 30 years) increasing the risk. Likewise, women who have never been pregnant are at higher risk. Breast feeding appears to protect against breast cancer.

3 Diet and alcohol

Diet and modest alcohol intake have also been implicated as contributory causes and, undoubtedly, diet plays a major, but as yet immeasurable, part in the risk of breast cancer. As research continues, more theories are developing concerning the role of fats in the diet and the influence of total calorie intake. The fact that the incidence of breast cancer is much lower in developing and Far Eastern countries where both fat and calorie intake are lower than in western societies would seem to give support to these theories.

4 Hormone replacement therapy

Hormone replacement therapy (HRT) probably increases the risk of breast cancer by about 40% above the average. It seems sensible to avoid HRT if there is a family history of breast cancer, that is a first-degree relative (mother, sister, daughter) affected by the disease; however, HRT can, overall, provide protection against many diseases.

5 The oral contraceptive pill

The contraceptive pill has long been controversial in its association with breast cancer and certainly progesterone-only pills appear to be perfectly safe. It is possible, however, that prolonged use of oestrogen-containing pills could slightly increase the risk of developing breast cancer.

6 Family history

Between 5 and 10% of all breast cancers are associated with significant genetic factors. The younger the onset of breast cancer the more likely it is to be genetic. One of the genes involved (BCRA1) has been identified on chromosome 17 and there is evidence for another breast cancer gene (BCRA2) on chromosome 13.

In the future, it may be possible to ascertain if affected members have an abnormal BRCA1 or -2 gene and then offer testing to unaffected family members. These tests will only be offered by clinics with highly-specialised genetic experts and counsellors as the tests may well generate considerable anxiety.

4 *Diagnosis and prognosis*

One of the features of breast cancer is that it may remain dormant for a long period of time. A small tumour may develop and remain virtually static before developing a more rapid growth pattern.

4.1 Basic features — signs and symptoms

About 80% of women with breast cancer first consult their doctor with a symptom that they notice themselves. The most common feature is a lump, but sometimes the nipple may have been drawn in or there is a slight puckering or swelling of the skin of the breast. There may be some discharge from the nipple. In those patients who do not recognise a symptom suggestive of breast cancer themselves, the signs may be found on examination for some other cause or on screening (see Section 4.4).

Characteristics

The breast swelling is usually hard with ill-defined outlines and is sometimes fixed to the muscles on the wall of the chest or to the skin over the breast. The nipple may appear to show signs resembling the skin disorder eczema. Rarely, the breast appears inflamed, but this occurs only in cases where the tumour has advanced rapidly. Lymph glands may be enlarged and this can be felt as lumps in the armpits.

4.2 Aims of diagnostic tests

Tests are designed to confirm the clinical diagnosis of breast cancer and to define the extent of disease in order to plan treatment.

Clinical examination

Clinical examination of the breast is only part of the procedure and rarely gives a definite diagnosis on its own. Even expert breast surgeons and oncologists (doctors who specialise in the treatment of cancer) do not diagnose whether a lump is benign or malignant on the basis of examination alone. A suspicious lump is usually subjected to an x-ray examination (mammography) and almost invariably a needle aspiration biopsy or full biopsy (described below) will be performed.

Needle aspiration biopsy

Needle aspiration biopsy is the removal of cellular material from a suspicious lump using an ordinary needle and syringe, perhaps using a small amount of local anaesthetic. This may be done in a clinic, perhaps with the assistance of a radiologist to locate the lump precisely and to ensure the correct tissue is sampled. Tiny amounts of material withdrawn through the needle are processed and examined by a pathologist to distinguish whether or not they are healthy. The pathologist will usually be able to say whether the cells detected are benign or malignant.

Breast biopsy

A breast biopsy, which provides a small piece of tissue for the pathologist to examine, may be carried out immediately or following needle aspiration biopsy. This procedure may not be necessary if the combination of clinical symptoms, signs, radiology results and cytology (the results of the needle aspiration) are absolutely convincing. However, most clinicians and pathologists prefer to confirm the diagnosis with a full biopsy as this gives a much fuller picture of the abnormal tissue as more cells are obtained. A full biopsy usually confirms the diagnosis of breast cancer.

If the mass of the abnormal tissue is large, a part may be removed before deciding on a treatment programme.

If the lump is small it may be totally removed, or excised, as part of the diagnostic procedure. As tissue removed in this way is processed by standardised pathology procedures, it may take two or three days to obtain a diagnosis. Part of the tissue may be sent off for special hormone tests to determine whether the presumed cancer is likely to be sensitive to hormone treatments (see Section 5).

Pathological diagnosis

A pathologist will be able to tell from a breast biopsy whether a breast lump is benign or malignant. A pathological diagnosis also allows the tumour to be classified. Different types of breast cancers have differing tendencies to spread; types that spread rapidly are termed 'aggressive' cancers and treatment must be planned accordingly.

Further surgical staging

The final procedure may be a surgical removal of some or all of the lymph glands in the underarm, known as axillary staging. Tumour cells detected within the lymph glands help define the risk of recurrence and the amount of treatment required.

Radiological tests

Mammography

A mammogram is an x-ray of the breast (see Figure 3). Mammography (see also Section 4.4) may help to define the extent of the tumour in the breast if the patient is strongly suspected of having breast cancer. It may show the surgeon that the lump can be removed without extensive tissue damage

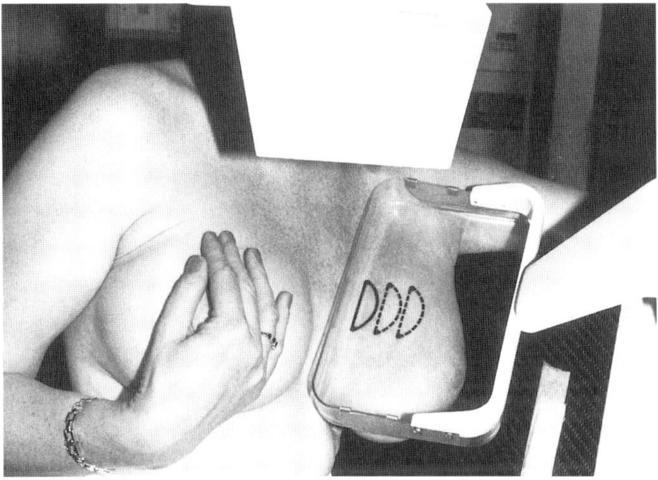

Figure 3. Breast examination using mammography

and may help to decide whether a full mastectomy (total removal of the breast) is necessary or whether an operation involving the more common procedure of removing the lump (lumpectomy), but conserving the breast, may be sufficient.

Ultrasound scanning

Ultrasound is being used more frequently for the diagnosis of breast cancer and treatment planning. It can, in some cases, be more effective than x-rays in determining the extent of the abnormal tissue in the breast.

Routine x-rays

Chest x-rays are performed routinely, before treatment is started, both to screen for the presence of secondary cancers in the lung and to check the general state of the heart and lungs before anaesthesia for surgery. Bone x-rays or isotope bone scans may be performed and, although they may be part of a routine 'screen' before surgery, are very likely to be performed on those patients with symptoms suggestive of secondary tumours outside the breast, particularly unexplained pain in the back or hips.

Other radiology

Computed tomography (CT) scanning and magnetic resonance imaging (MRI) scanning are increasingly being used in the management of all malignant diseases, with breast cancer being no exception. Both techniques are useful for examining sites deep within the body, including the spinal cord and the brain. The main disadvantage is that some patients find the long narrow tunnel design of the scanner claustrophobic. However, MRI unlike all the other radiology diagnostic tests, with the exception of ultrasound, is considered to be safe because there is no actual radiation involved in obtaining the images.

Carcinoma in situ
Pathological tests may distinguish the cancer as being carcinoma *in situ*, where it appears to be confined to the breast ducts or lobules and has no immediate tendency to spread outside the breast. National studies are being conducted to determine the best method of treatment for this type of cancer.

4.3 What is secondary breast cancer? How does cancer spread?

The spread of tumour cells from one organ to another, not directly connected with it, is known as metastasis and results in secondary cancers (metastases or secondaries). Figure 4 depicts the sequence of events in metastasis.

As shown in Figure 4, metastasis involves the following:

- release of cells from the original malignant tumour, usually referred to as the primary tumour;
- the spread of these cells to distant parts of the body via the lymphatic system (usually through the lymph glands in the armpits), the blood stream or by infiltrating the tissues in the original site to produce skin secondaries; and

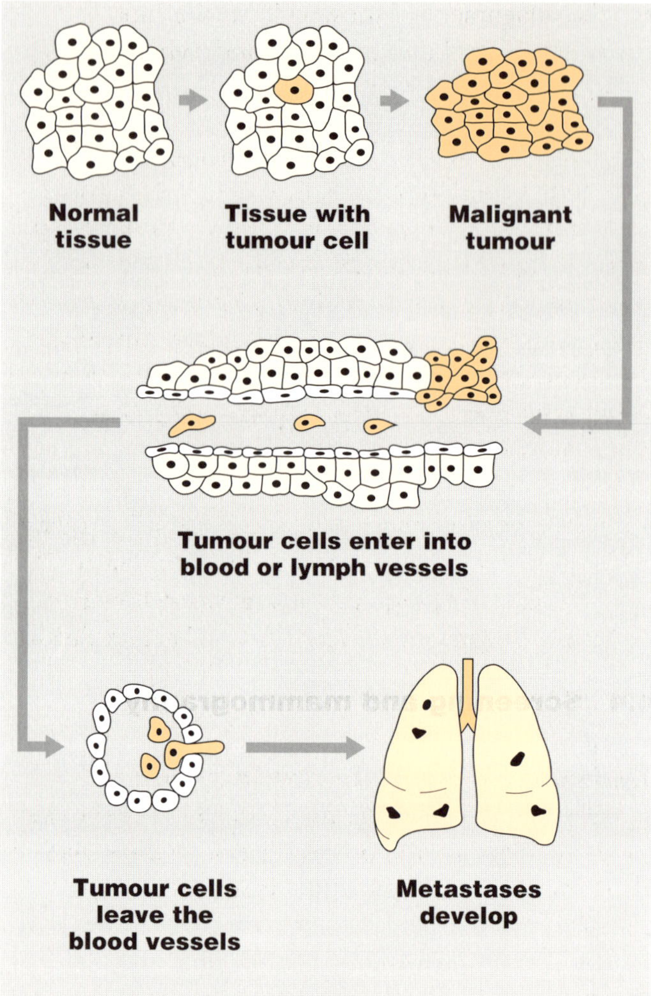

Figure 4. Spread of cancer (metastasis)

- the attachment of these cells to the blood vessels and the organs involved, whereafter they grow into new tumours.

Secondary tumours of breast cancer appear to be common in the lymph glands, particularly those in the armpit near the affected breast, in the lungs (or in the linings of the lungs, the pleura), liver, bones, skin and sometimes in the brain. The cells that spread do not always form a secondary cancer as soon as they have lodged themselves in another location: they may die or lie dormant for years before becoming active again.

Secondary breast cancer can manifest itself in many ways depending on the organs that are affected. It is a condition that requires separate consideration and it is not appropriate to discuss it here in detail.

4.4 Screening and mammography

The key to early detection of breast cancer is screening, that is looking for cancer in women who have no obvious symptoms of disease. Early detection also requires breast self-examination (see pages 26–28).

Results of studies in Scandinavia, North America and the United Kingdom have led to the conclusion that breast screening, based on the use of mammography, should be adopted as a national policy for women between the ages of 50 and 64 years. Women in this age bracket are at relatively high risk of developing breast cancer and mammography provides good images of abnormal lumps with a 95% chance of an accurate diagnosis.

Mammography can detect a lump as much as two years before it can be felt and cancers found in this way are smaller and may not have spread. The majority of cancers that are too small to be felt can be removed totally.

Figure 5 emphasises the importance of early detection of breast cancer by breast self-examination and screening.

Screening units are run by expert radiologists and breast surgeons. Any suspicious signs detected are investigated further by referral for diagnostic tests (see Section 4.2). However, the breasts of younger women tend to be somewhat more dense, radiologically, such that mammography is less useful in this age group.

Now that a gene associated with a large proportion of inherited breast cancer has been identified, it will be possible to screen younger women with a strong family history of breast cancer. Genetic counselling

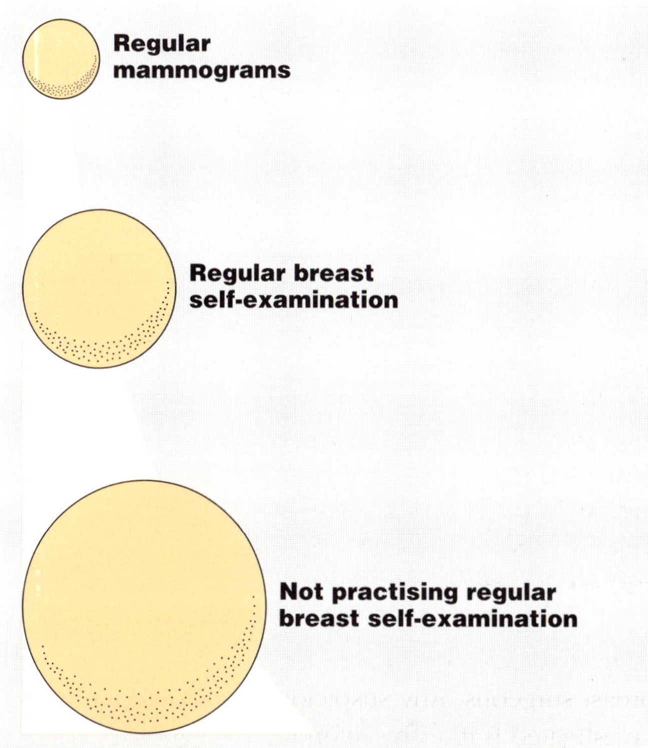

Figure 5. Representation of the size of tumours detected by various methods

clinics are being established in some areas of the United Kingdom to advise women with such family histories and to screen, with techniques available currently, those family members thought to be at highest risk.

Breast awareness

Breast awareness is the process of getting to know your breasts and finding what is normal for you.

When you know how your breasts look and feel normally, you will be the first to notice any changes (see Figures 6 and 7).

You should look for any changes in your breast that are unusual for you in terms of normal shape and size, normal appearance and position of your nipples and the normal 'feel' of your breasts. Figures 6 and 7 will direct you towards checking your breasts by looking and feeling.

If you find any changes, seek medical advice immediately.

You may find self-examination easier if you follow a particular pattern using the flat of your hand and the fingertips, moving the fingers in up-and-down lines or strips. Try using a circular motion or moving your fingers in 'wedges' starting at the outer edge of the breast, moving towards the nipple and out again. Check the whole breast, one 'wedge' at a time. Develop a routine, but cover all the breast, up to the collar bone and to the underarm area, including the armpits.

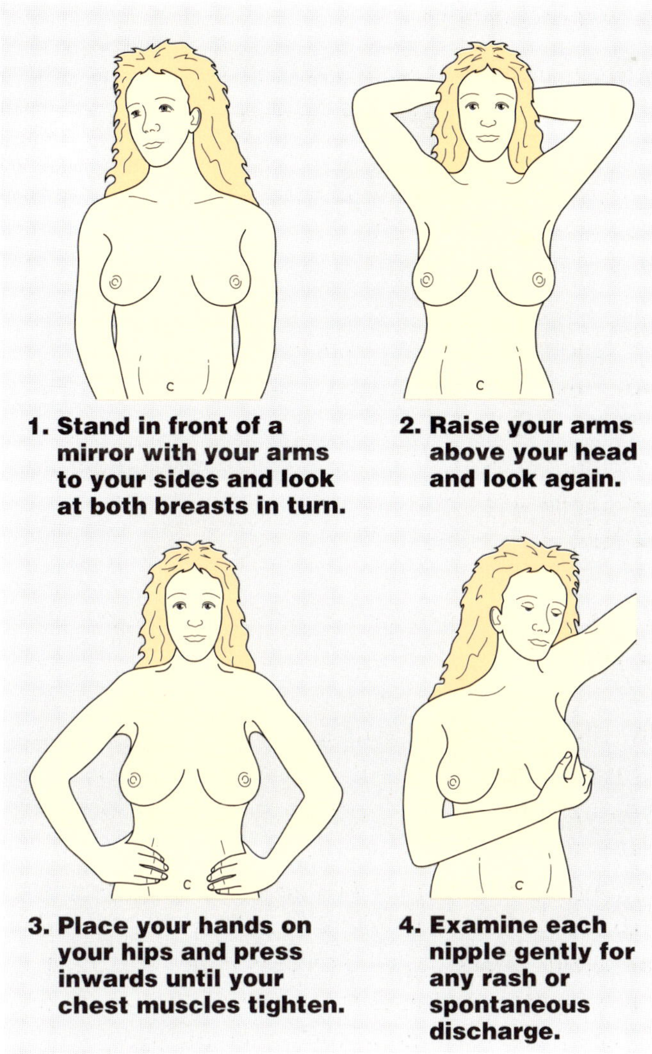

Figure 6. Breast awareness — looking

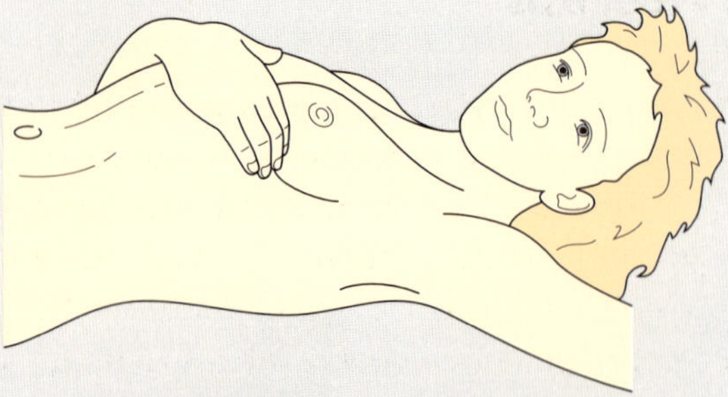

1. Feel your breast in the bath or shower with a soapy hand or, for those with larger breasts, when lying on a bed.

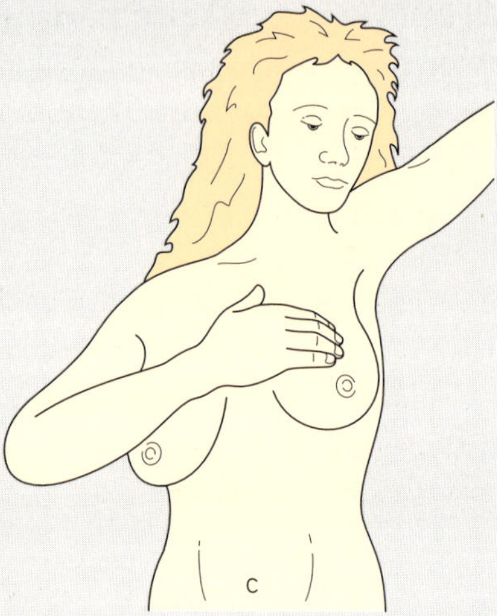

2. Keep your fingers together and use the flat of the hand and fingertips. Press the breast gently, but firmly, by moving your fingers over the whole breast.

Figure 7. Breast awareness — feeling

4. 5 Prognosis

The term prognosis means the expert opinion of the probable course and outcome of an illness based upon all the relevant, attainable facts of the case. All findings from clinical examinations and radiological investigations are thus important and must be considered together to decide what the progress of an individual case of breast cancer is likely to be. From this, the most appropriate course of treatment can be decided and put into action. However, the treatment strategy chosen will vary from patient to patient and the various treatments available are discussed in the next section. With prompt and appropriate treatment, the outlook for a woman with breast cancer can be good.

In particular, the surgeon or oncologist will be looking for some very specific features in the newly-diagnosed cancer, before pronouncing on its likely behaviour and thus how to treat it to prevent complications. The main features are:

1 Are the local (underarm) lymph nodes involved, and if so, how many? Have the nodes been 'sampled' or totally removed and examined microscopically?

2 How big is the breast cancer?

3 What special features are seen in the 'primary' cancer? Are the microscopic blood vessels or lymph channels invaded?

4 Do the cancer cells in the breast look 'aggressive'?

5 Is the tumour safely removable by surgery, ie is the skin involved? Are other sites in the body invaded?

5 *Treatment of breast cancer*

The main aim of current treatment, after preserving life, is to conserve the breast as far as possible, unless the patient herself elects for a mastectomy. It has long been proven that radical mastectomy (total removal of the affected breast and chest wall muscles) alone cannot cure the majority of breast cancers. More emphasis is now placed on causing the least damage possible with local treatment, ie of the breast area alone and by the increasing use of 'systemic' treatment, ie treatment for the whole body with chemotherapy or hormone therapy to prevent recurrence.

There are some patients in whom it may not be possible to conserve the breast, in which case a mastectomy is required. However, a good cosmetic result can be often achieved with the help of reconstructive surgery and possibly the use of silicone implants and tissue expanders.

If breast conservation is to be a satisfactory and efficient treatment for an individual patient, the following requirements have to be considered:

- It must be possible to perform adequate surgery to remove the malignant lump, but to preserve most of the breast tissue.

- It must be possible to obtain sufficient material from the axillary lymph nodes (those in the armpit) to obtain an accurate prognosis.
- 'Radical' radiotherapy must be applied to the disease site and to the remaining breast tissue. This may include radiation of the axilla (armpit), but depends on the extent of the surgery performed previously.
- These treatments should be combined with appropriate 'adjuvant' (or additional/ complementary) systemic treatment. 'Systemic' treatment is treatment applied to the whole body; in contrast, 'local' treatment is applied only to the site of disease. Radiotherapy can be local, but hormonal treatment and chemotherapy (drugs given by mouth or by injection) are systemic. Chemotherapy and hormone therapy can contribute significantly towards reducing the risk of breast cancer recurrence in patients of all ages.

5.1 Surgery

Surgery is performed in order to obtain the best local control of the disease. If this is not performed adequately, there is an increased risk of the cancer returning or recurring, either locally, ie at the site of the original tumour, or nearby. This is the major concern of surgeons and radiotherapists when deciding an individual's suitability for breast conservation treatment. For example, patients who have several tumour sites in the breast may not be suitable for conservation treatment and those who have tumours very near the skin or at the very edge of the breast may also not be suitable.

Patients who have small breasts and relatively large lumps may not have a good cosmetic appearance after partial removal of a breast and may obtain a better final appearance from having a mastectomy and reconstruction procedure. Widespread involvement of the lymph system in the breast also counts against conservation procedures. After taking the advice of the pathologist, who examines the tissue removed during an attempt at a conservation procedure, the surgeon may decide to remove more tissue or to perform a mastectomy.

Age should not be a major factor in deciding the suitability of breast conservation.

With the advent of mammography screening, breast cancers are being detected early, ie before they can be detected as lumps. These small growths can be removed successfully by surgery by using radiology to locate them accurately and to check for complete removal.

5.2 Post-operative treatment

The treatment that is given after surgery (post-operative treatment) is designed to minimise the risk of cancer recurring. The following treatments are usually considered.

Radiotherapy

Modern, high-energy radiotherapy may be necessary in case any cancer cells remain in the breast or lymph glands. Radiotherapy should provide satisfactory treatment without producing unacceptable tissue damage when used accurately and in appropriate doses. Treatment is usually given over three to five weeks in 15–20 'fractions' or individual treatments. Top-up doses may be given later using electron therapy or sometimes by inserting radioactive wires into the tissue from which the cancer was removed. Radiotherapy to the axilla is not normally recommended if full axillary dissection has been undertaken.

It is known that the combination of breast conserving surgery and radiotherapy is as good as radical mastectomy (complete removal of the breast and chest wall muscles) for the control of breast cancer in appropriately selected cases. Whether or not to apply radiotherapy to the armpit is a matter for discussion between the surgeon and radiotherapists and depends on the amount of tissue removed at surgery and the extent to which the lymph nodes in the armpit are involved as determined by the pathologist.

Irradiation of the armpit is not routine because excessive damage to the tissues in this area from surgery and radiotherapy can lead to blockage of the lymph channels with unpleasant swelling and discomfort in the arm.

Breast reconstruction

Any patient who has had a mastectomy should be offered the chance of a reconstruction to achieve the best cosmetic result as this may have a considerable impact on the patient's feelings about the operation. The necessary surgery may be performed by a specialist breast surgeon, a plastic surgeon or both. Surgery may be performed more or less immediately after mastectomy or may be delayed until after radiotherapy or chemotherapy. Some surgeons recommend delaying surgery for six months.

An inflatable tissue expander may be used at the site of mastectomy to prepare for the eventual insertion of a permanent silicone implant.

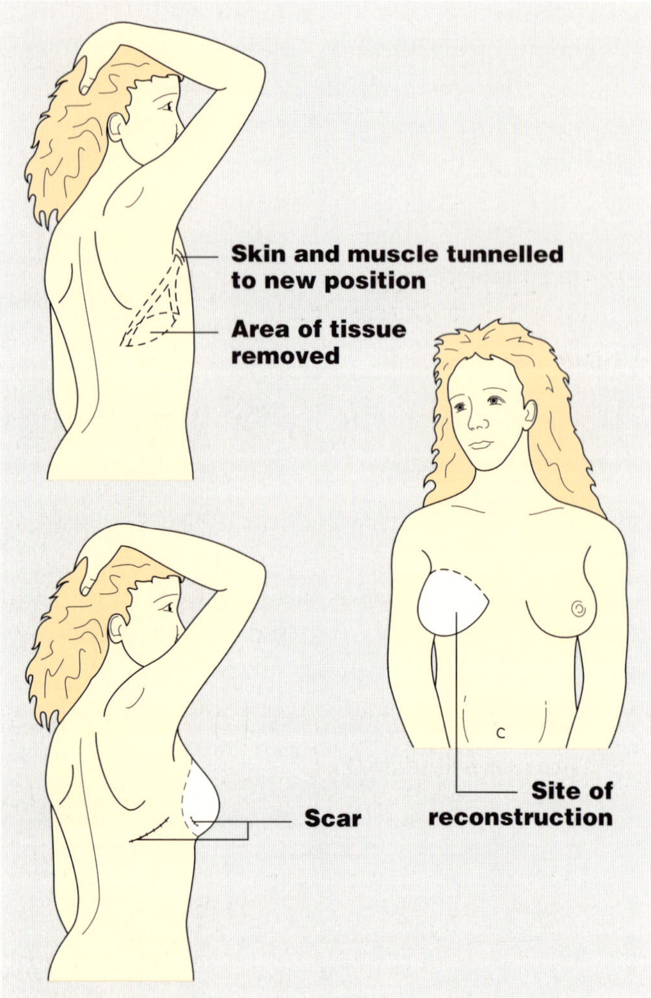

Figure 8. Breast reconstruction — using muscle from the back

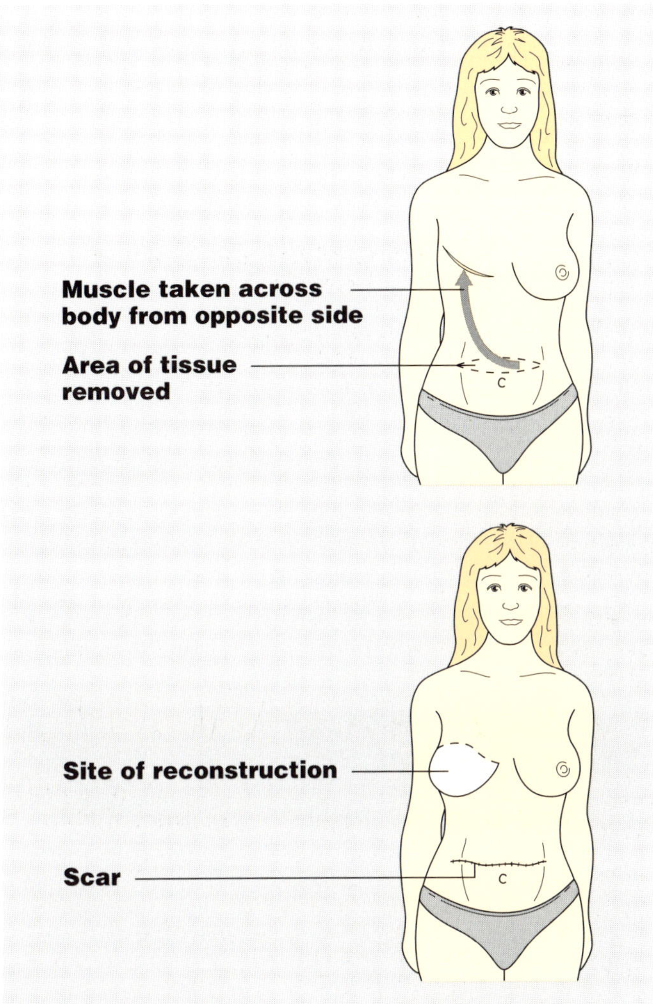

Figure 9. Breast reconstruction — using muscle from the abdomen

This insertion does not increase the risk of a second cancer. It is also important to know that, despite legal proceedings in the United States, there are no proven serious complications arising from the use of silicone implants.

Alternatively, the area under the mastectomy scar can be built up with the patient's own fat and muscle, which is taken from the back (an 'L D flap') or from the wall of the abdomen (a 'Tram flap') (see Figures 8 and 9). A nipple reconstruction can be very acceptable cosmetically, but most patients are happy enough to regain their breast outline only.

Despite similar surgical techniques, results can vary from one patient to the next. It is important for the surgeon and patient to discuss the worst as well as the best cosmetic results of breast conserving surgery.

Hormonal treatment

In 1896 a surgeon, George Beatson, showed that hormone treatment could influence human cancer. His reasoning was that breast cancer was likely to be a hormone-dependent tumour and that by removing the ovaries, the main source of the female hormone oestrogen, cancer regression would occur. This proved to be correct in two cases of advanced disease.

In the subsequent 100 years of breast cancer treatment, a variety of approaches to hormone treatment have been used and these are listed in Table 1.

About two-thirds of advanced breast cancer patients with hormone-dependent tumours will respond to hormone treatments within an average of 12–18 months. Selecting therapy to influence hormone levels depends on the side-effects of treatment.

Table 1. Hormone treatments

1	Removal of ovaries (ovariectomy) for pre-menopausal patients. Reversible ovary blockade with drugs (for example, Zoladex®, Zeneca Pharma) and instead of or preliminary to removal of the ovaries.
2	Using anti-oestrogen compounds, such as tamoxifen (Nolvadex®, Zeneca Pharma; Tamofen™, Pharmacia Ltd; Emblon®, Berk Pharmaceuticals Ltd and Oestrifen®, Ashbourne Pharmaceuticals Ltd)
3	Using progestogens (other female hormones) in high doses
4	Using compounds known as 'synthesis inhibitors', including drugs that block the

production of oestrogen. These drugs are taken as tablets or given by injection. Using compounds that inhibit the enzyme 'aromatase' which is important in production of oestrogen after the menopause

Pituitary and adrenal surgery and the use of other hormones have largely disappeared from practice because of perceived complications or other toxicities.

With the advent of modern drugs, virtually all methods of hormone therapy that involve surgery, apart from ovariectomy, have been abandoned.

Current use of hormone therapy is based, therefore, on one of the following, more limited, range of treatments.

Anti-oestrogens (tamoxifen)

Tamoxifen is the routine breast cancer hormone therapy and is used for both pre- and post-menopausal patients. This drug is a potent inhibitor of oestrogen stimulation of breast cancer and is successful because it effectively blocks the action of oestrogen on the tumour and, generally, has a very low rate of significant side-effects. Occasionally a patient may experience hot flushes, vaginal bleeding and vaginal discharge resulting from mildly hormone-stimulating effects on the vagina. However, any patient experiencing vaginal bleeding should consult their doctor so that other possible causes are identified. Patients may also experience some nausea, skin rash and light-headedness.

Tamoxifen is easy to take as a tablet and probably has some beneficial effects in having oestrogenic protective effects on the bone against osteoporosis (brittle bones) and the heart against middle-aged coronary heart disease. One potential drawback to its use is the slightly increased risk of cancer of the womb (uterine cancer). This is recognised as a potential problem and can be watched for, diagnosed early and treated effectively. It should be remembered that the number of lives saved through the use of tamoxifen vastly exceeds the number of complications caused by its use.

Progestogens

One or two of these compounds [for example, medroxyprogesterone acetate (Depo-Provera® and Provera®, Upjohn Ltd and Farlutal®, Pharmacia Ltd) and megestrol acetate (Megace®, Bristol-Myers Squibb Pharmaceuticals)] are very effective as second-line treatments for breast cancer after tamoxifen has failed or if, for some unusual reason, tamoxifen is not well tolerated. The effectiveness and side-effects of progestogens are similar to those of tamoxifen, with one of the side-effects being fluid retention. Patients taking progestogens may also experience weight gain as a result of appetite stimulation. Patients with impaired heart function may be at particular risk of developing fluid retention and may require diuretics to control this effect.

In post-menopausal patients, prolonged use of progestogens can lead to vaginal bleeding. Any unusual vaginal bleeding needs to be investigated by a gynaecologist to confirm that there is no problem other than the side-effects of treatment.

Aromatase inhibitors

Aromatase inhibitors are currently in use for the treatment of post-menopausal breast cancer. They act by blocking the production of oestrogen.

Aminoglutethimide (Orimeten®, Ciba Pharmaceuticals) is taken by mouth (usually with hydrocortisone). Although, aminoglutethimide is an effective treatment, some patients experience side-effects such as skin rash and drowsiness. These side-effects are far less common with newer aromatase inhibitors such as formestane (Lentaron®, Ciba Pharmaceuticals). Formestane is administered by injection every two weeks and it is not necessary to take additional hydrocortisone. Formestane blocks oestrogen production more specifically than aminoglutethimide and side-effects are generally less of a problem.

Recent developments in this area have produced some drugs that are effective after tamoxifen no longer controls the cancer. They are particularly attractive because they produce very few side-effects. Anastrazole (Arimidex®, Zeneca) became available in late 1995 and is given as a single dose at 1mg daily and so is easy to administer. Other compounds of this type are expected.

Pituitary suppressants

These drugs have to be given by injection or by nasal spray and are therefore rather inconvenient; however, a monthly 'depot' dosage scheme is possible, making administration less difficult for patients. However, these drugs are expensive, require repeated administration and are probably inferior to the procedure of ovariectomy, particularly since the latter can now be performed simply through a laparoscope. Nevertheless, these drugs may be used to test for the usefulness of surgery in a patient with symptomatic advanced disease: if a patient responds to therapy over a few months with a pituitary suppressant, it may be worthwhile proceeding to ovariectomy as the definitive procedure.

Ovariectomy

Ovariectomy (or oöphorectomy) is the removal of the ovaries. As this procedure reduces the risk of recurrence from breast cancer in younger patients, it is recommended as a useful treatment for certain types of pre-menopausal breast cancer. Patients who seem to have hormone-sensitive tumours appear to be good candidates for this procedure. It is unclear how best to use ovariectomy and chemotherapy and current trials are examining whether ovariectomy and chemotherapy should be used together or separately. For the treatment of advanced disease, however, drug treatments tend to be preferred to ovariectomy.

Chemotherapy

Chemotherapy as an adjuvant treatment for primary breast cancer

Cancer cells may, in some patients, spread to other

parts of the body before surgery has been performed. However, in most cases only microscopic numbers of cancer cells (if any) have spread by the time surgery is performed and these are not detectable by even the most sensitive scan. 'Adjuvant' therapy aims to eradicate these cells before they have a chance to grow and become obvious secondary deposits. Two main types of adjuvant therapy are used in the treatment of breast cancer:

1. **Chemotherapy** — to kill cancer cells
2. **Hormone therapy** — to deprive cancer cells of the hormones that are required for their survival.

The place of chemotherapy in the treatment of breast cancer is now established as a means of preventing disease recurrence. For example, if the lymph glands are affected by cancer in a younger patient, chemotherapy may be the best additional treatment to surgery and radiotherapy. Chemotherapy is given routinely for four to six months and may precede or follow radiotherapy. It may also be used alongside radiotherapy following local surgery.

Some interesting results have been obtained from the use of chemotherapy as a first treatment for breast cancer, that is primary chemotherapy. It is being found that, in many cases, chemotherapy can shrink breast tumours prior to surgery. This approach to treatment may help to minimise further the surgery required (avoiding mastectomy) and may reduce the risk of later recurrence. This method is currently under trial in several hospitals.

The standard adjuvant chemotherapy treatment involves three drugs [cyclophosphamide (Endoxana®, ASTA Medica Ltd), methotrexate (methotrexate™, American Cyanamid Co; Maxtrex®, Pharmacia Ltd), 5-fluorouracil (Fluoro-Uracil Roche®, Roche Products Limited)] and is known as the CMF chemotherapy regimen. This treatment sometimes causes nausea and fatigue, but significant hair loss is not usually a feature. Using this combination is certainly better than using one drug alone, as was common in the 1970s, in preventing recurrence. Other combinations used in the treatment of breast cancer are shown in Table 2.

Chemotherapy for advanced disease

Chemotherapy for the treatment of advanced breast cancer is an area of great controversy in almost every respect. If breast cancer recurs, it is treated routinely with hormone therapy for as long as possible as this form of therapy causes fewer side-effects and yet can produce the most long-lasting remissions. Unfortunately, across the whole population of patients with recurrent disease, hormone therapy will only produce useful disease regression in about 30% of patients, with another

Table 2. Combination chemotherapy regimens used in the treatment of breast cancer

• **CMF**	cyclophosphamide methotrexate 5-fluorouracil
• **MMM**	mitozantrone (Novantrone®, Lederle Laboratories) methotrexate mitomycin C
• **FAC**	5-fluorouracil doxorubicin cyclophosphamide
• **ECF**	epirubicin (Pharmorubicin®, Pharmacia Ltd) platinum infusional 5-FU
• **CMFVP**	cyclophosphamide methotrexate 5-fluorouracil vincristine (Oncovin®, Lilly Eli & Co. Ltd) prednisolone

Paclitaxel (Taxol™, Bristol-Myers Squibb Pharmaceuticals), docetaxel (Taxotere®, Rhône-Poulenc Rorer Ltd) and idarubicin (Zavedos®, Pharmacia Ltd) show promise in early trials.

approximately 20% having so-called disease stabilisation for a period. This means that more than 50% of patients so treated will not respond usefully and will require chemotherapy to obtain control of their disease. However, chemotherapy will rarely cure advanced breast cancer, but can certainly reduce symptoms and almost certainly prolongs the survival of some patients with life-threatening complications. The main problem is that the effectiveness of the chemotherapy is broadly related to the intensity with which it is given so that most side-effects are associated with treatments that are most effective in terms of tumour regression.

There are therefore roughly two options regarding the administration of chemotherapy:

1 To produce minimal side-effects, but a reasonable number of tumour regressions.
2 To apply more aggressive therapy to produce a maximum degree of control and to accept the higher level of chemotherapy-associated side-effects (see Section 6).

Several developments have occurred recently in the field of chemotherapy for advanced breast cancer. A new class of compounds called the taxoids is proving useful being effective after doxorubicin has failed to control disease. However, because of their high level of activity they are also being used in initial treatment of advanced disease, either alone or increasingly in combination with other drugs.

The selection of treatment may be determined partly by factors such as the patient's age and general fitness. There is therefore a slight tendency to use more aggressive therapy for younger patients with major symptoms such as liver damage or lung damage from secondary tumours. In contrast, an elderly patient who has progression of disease on hormone therapy may be offered gentle chemotherapy to try to relieve symptoms.

It is important to recognise that the outlook for breast cancer is influenced only partly by the treatment applied. Thus, a patient who has 'grumbling disease' involving the lymph glands, skin or even bones tends to respond rather better in the long-term than a patient who has impairment of liver or lung function due to metastases. Similarly, patients with secondary tumours in the brain will succumb very quickly to the tumour unless effective radiation treatment can arrest the disease progression, but even then the effect of treatment is usually only temporary.

The choice of chemotherapy therefore involves separate judgement for individual cases and a wide variety of chemical agents have been tried in different combinations and treatment schemes.

5.3 Non-surgical management of breast cancer

Between 10 and 15% of patients with breast cancer cannot be operated upon at the time of first diagnosis. This may be because the tumour is growing very rapidly or because there has been a delay in diagnosing breast cancer. In an elderly patient, radiotherapy may be the best treatment option in order to gain control of the tumour locally. Primary medical treatment with chemotherapy or hormone therapy without previous surgery will delay or prevent recurrence at other sites.

Younger patients are generally offered chemotherapy and older patients hormone therapy in an attempt to reduce the size of the tumour before radiotherapy is used. Very dramatic reductions in tumour size can be achieved with quite intensive chemotherapy and surgery becomes a possibility in about one-third of such cases. This surgery may be performed before or after radiotherapy, depending on the individual case.

6 *Management of the side-effects associated with treatment for breast cancer*

Different chemotherapy agents cause different side-effects, but the following appear to be common to most chemotherapy treatments.

6.1 Fatigue

Fatigue is common and hard to deal with, particularly in patients who are otherwise well, for example patients who are given adjuvant chemotherapy following surgery for a primary tumour. Patients with advanced disease who are ill from the effects of cancer may find that the annoyance of fatigue from chemotherapy is outweighed by an improvement in their symptoms.

6.2 Nausea and vomiting

Nausea and vomiting was once the major complication of chemotherapy, but can be controlled largely by the use of a variety of antisickness drugs, either alone or in combination. Some antisickness drugs are expensive and may be reserved for patients who have had bad experiences with chemotherapy previously.

Some patients may experience nausea and vomiting even before chemotherapy is given — this is known as 'anticipatory nausea and vomiting' and may be controlled by mild sedatives before a hospital visit. These symptoms can be usually controlled by an injection at the time of chemotherapy and by taking tablets at home for the first 24–48 hours post-treatment. Symptoms after this time are unusual.

6.3 Hair loss

Treatment of advanced disease with more potent chemotherapy agents almost routinely causes hair loss and the patient will be made aware of this and receive counselling. Hair loss is not immediate and the hair always grows back. A wig should be provided through the health service, but a small financial contribution may have to be made by the patient.

6.4 Menopausal symptoms

Chemotherapy suppresses the function of the ovaries such that prolonged or intensive chemotherapy is likely, particularly in older pre-menopausal patients (those over 40 years), to suppress oestrogen production by the ovaries. In this case, the patient develops menopausal symptoms. The normal function of the ovaries may or may not return after chemotherapy is completed, but is more likely to do so in younger patients. In any event, chemotherapy seems to bring forward the age of the menopause by several years.

6.5 Haematological (blood) complications

Chemotherapy may have serious effects on the immune system although treatments are designed to cause as few disruptions as possible. Chemotherapy can reduce the number of white cells — the cells that help fight infection in the blood — making the patient susceptible to infection by bacteria. The risk is highest seven to ten days after chemotherapy when the patient is at risk of developing pneumonia, which can be very serious if not treated promptly. The patient and her doctor should be aware of the need for expert diagnosis and treatment at this time. Having said this, most patients go through months of chemotherapy without experiencing this complication.

7 *Complications of breast cancer*

7.1 Local disease and ulceration

Local disease and ulceration is one of the most unpleasant complications of breast cancer, but is quite uncommon provided that the disease is diagnosed before it spreads locally, that is within the breast. It may be relieved partly by radiation treatment or by drug therapy. A persistent ulcer will probably become infected and local dressing and antibiotics will be needed to relieve the symptoms.

7.2 Bone secondaries

The bones are a common site of breast cancer recurrence, that is development of a secondary cancer after the primary tumour has been removed surgically. However, active treatment can be very satisfactory and the disease can be controlled with simple hormonal therapy. A woman can have years of active life with bone secondaries. However, pain may be a problem and a variety of pain killers or local radiotherapy may be required.

Occasionally the hip bone can threaten to break due to weakening of this weight-bearing bone because of secondary cancer and an orthopaedic operation may be required to strengthen the area prior to pain-relieving radiotherapy.

Multiple secondary cancers in the bones may need chemotherapy to control disease and in some patients damage to the skeleton as a result of disease may lead to hypercalcaemia (raised levels of calcium in the blood). This can lead to complications unless treated promptly with a specific drug.

7.3 Cough and shortness of breath

Symptoms of coughing and shortness of breath may mean that the disease is affecting the lungs by causing a build-up of fluid on the lungs (pleural effusion) or may be due to direct damage to the lungs (infiltration). The effusion may be drained easily using a needle inserted between the ribs or through a soft, thin drainage catheter. Sometimes a drug needs to be instilled into the pleural cavity (the space around the lungs) to prevent recurrence. Ultimately, control of lung disease requires effective systemic hormone therapy or chemotherapy.

7.4 Lymphoedema

Lymphoedema is the presence of excessive amounts of fluid in the lymph system (the lymphatic channels and lymph glands). This can manifest as swelling of the arm after surgery or radiotherapy because the drainage of the lymph from the arm is inadequate due to damage in the underarm lymph nodes (axillary). A pressure bandage or stocking may help to reduce the amount of swelling and the assistance of a physiotherapist can be important.

7.5 Fatigue and weight loss

Fatigue and weight loss often occur as a temporary reaction to chemotherapy. However, these symptoms may, in a patient with advanced cancer, indicate that cancer has spread to the liver and that urgent drug treatment is required, possibly with steroids and probably chemotherapy.

8 *Psychological aspects*

8.1 Adjusting to the diagnosis and primary treatment

It is common for an individual to become anxious and depressed after a diagnosis of cancer, especially in younger patients and those with previous psychological difficulties. Studies have shown that around 30% of patients consistently require specific counselling, preferably from a nurse with special training. Not surprisingly, mastectomy itself causes psychological trauma as do radiotherapy and chemotherapy. There is no increase in anxiety for patients undergoing mastectomy, but problems with body image are common. There is very little evidence to show the effects of radiotherapy and chemotherapy on the occurrence of anxiety and depression.

All the treatments discussed in this book are traumatic in different ways and, used together, mean that, mentally as well as physically, the patient goes through a testing time, sometimes over a period of many months before their treatment is completed. The addition of long-term hormone treatment to prevent recurrence may be easy enough to cope with physically but, again, mentally serves to remind the patient of the risk of recurrence.

There is no substitute for careful counselling, in the general sense, from all staff involved with the patient; it is important that the patient understands that a team of carers is often essential.

There seems little doubt that the patient's attitude to the disease and its treatment are profoundly influenced by the first consultation when the diagnosis is made. Many doctors now recognise the advantage of consulting with the patient supported by her family, usually her husband or partner, who can minimise the patient's sense of isolation. A supportive partner may also recall details about the prognosis and treatment that the patient, in a distressed and possibly confused state, may misunderstand or forget.

8.2 The patient's emotions and reactions

Even with the best support, the patient may need a long time to accept the situation. Anger, shock and even denial are normal reactions to bad news and, when the strong cultural and sexual connotations of the illness are added to these reactions, it is hardly surprising that breast cancer is a challenge not only to the patient, but to family, friends and professional carers alike. Given that both hormonal therapy and chemotherapy can induce early menopausal symptoms in younger patients, this adds yet another level of stress.

8.3 The problems of very advanced disease and terminal illness

All of the above traumas are amplified for the patient who has to face the onset of recurrent and possibly far advanced disease. Although it may be generally recognised both by staff and patients that a recurrence of breast cancer is rarely curable, it is important to stress that a patient may have many years of active life. An accurate appraisal of the prognosis requires expert knowledge and may require careful investigation of the extent of disease to provide the necessary information to the patient who truly wishes to know how the disease is likely to progress.

For other patients, denial of the prognosis can be a reasonable and effective way of coping with the situation. For such a patient, who is perhaps basically 'well', excessive investigation and tests can be counter-productive.

Most doctors and nurses find the process of disclosing bad news very difficult. Much depends on the personalities of the staff as well as that of the patient and their preceding relationship. Sharing of information should, perhaps, be a gradual process, and a trained and sensitive carer will recognise how much a patient wants to know at any given time.

9 *Support groups and counselling*

It is important that any woman with breast cancer realises that she is not alone. There are cancer support and self-help groups throughout the United Kingdom and all over the world. There are also many local groups and information should be available from doctor's surgeries or from directories at local libraries. The following national associations will give emotional support and practical help to a woman with breast cancer or to her friends and relatives.

Breast Cancer Care

Breast Cancer Care (BCC, formerly known as the Breast Care and Mastectomy Association of Great Britain or BCMA) offers free help, information and support to women with breast cancer or other breast-related problems. Its services include help and information lines, a range of information leaflets on aspects of breast care and information on how to obtain a prosthesis (artificial breast), both on the NHS and through retail outlets. The organisation itself is able to supply prostheses and has fitting facilities in London, Glasgow and Edinburgh. This association offers advice on clothing and swimwear and arranges fashion shows around the country.

In addition, the BCC helpline will answer any queries with practical information and has trained volunteer helpers with experience of breast cancer and a nurse who can offer medical advice.

BCC help and information lines:

London	0171-867 1103
Glasgow	0141-353 1050
Edinburgh	0131-221 0407
Fax	0171-867 9303

Free Helpline (sponsored by Nationwide Building Society)	0500-245 345

BCC can be contacted by letter at : Breast Cancer Care, 15–19 Britten Street, London SW3 3TZ *or* Suite 2/8, 65 Bath Street, Glasgow G2 2BX.

Womens Nationwide Cancer Control Campaign (WNCCC)

The main aims of this campaign are early detection and prevention and a nationwide clinic list is maintained so that that any woman can find the facilities nearest to her. Their helpline provides information and emotional support on breast screening. The emphasis is on screening and WNCCC does not deal with queries about established cancer or its treatment. Literature is free to individual women, is available in 10 languages and can be obtained by writing to: Womens Nationwide Cancer Control Campaign, Suna House, 128 Curtain Road, London EC2A 3ARE.

Helpline:	0171-729 2229

CancerLink

CancerLink is for any individual with cancer, not just women with breast cancer. CancerLink is used by cancer patients as well as their families and friends and professionals working with them. Information is provided by telephone and letter (**CancerLink**, 17 Britannia Street, London WC1X 9JN *or* 9 Castle Terrace, Edinburgh EH1 2DP).

Their information service can offer support and information and helps clarify the treatment options available enabling more informed decisions to be made.

Telephone information lines	
London	0171-833 2451
Edinburgh	0131-228 5557
Asian language information and support line (Hindi, Bengali, Gujerati, Punjabi, Urdu and Cantonese)	0171-713 7867

A range of booklets that discuss cancer and its emotional impact are available and CancerLink will put individuals with cancer in touch with cancer support and self-help groups in their vicinity through The Group Support Service.

British Association of Cancer United Patients

The British Association of Cancer United Patients (BACUP) gives advice and information about all aspects of cancer as well as emotional support for individuals affected by breast cancer and their families and friends. Their Cancer Information Service is staffed by a team of specially trained nurses and supported by a panel of medical specialists. BACUP's Cancer Counselling service is available to anyone who can travel to the London or Glasgow office. They can also help individuals to find a counselling service if they live in another part of the country. Write to **BACUP** at 3 Bath Place, Rivington Street, London EC2A 3JR.

Cancer information service:	
From London	0171-613 2121
From outside London	Freeline: 0800 181199

Counselling service	
London	0171-696 9000
Glasgow	0141-248 9277

Cancer Care Society

The Cancer Care Society (CARE) offers counselling, emotional support and practical information, rather than medical support, for patients and their families and friends. They have a network of nationwide support groups run for and by individuals with direct experience of cancer. This society also has telephone link arrangements for individual support, arranging contact between enquirers and those in their own area with similar experiences. Write to **CARE** at 21 Zetland Road, Redland, Bristol BS6 7A.

Telephone:	0117-942 7419

Cancer Relief Macmillan Nurses

Clearly the advent of hospices, palliative care specialists (those who treat patients to minimise the symptoms of life-threatening diseases) and Macmillan Cancer Care Nurses has been of great value in educating surgeons and oncologists as well as providing effective care for the patient both in the hospital and community. There are a number of Macmillan Breast Cancer Nurses based in hospitals and a women with breast cancer can be referred by her general practitioner to one of these specialist nurses right from the point of diagnosis and at any stage of her illness. The nurse will provide emotional support, practical information and advice from initial diagnosis throughout treatment. Most of these nurses work in conjunction with a team that specialises in breast cancer.

Macmillan Breast Cancer Nurses can be contacted by writing to: **Cancer Relief Macmillan Fund**, 15–19 Britten Street, London SW3 3TZ.

Telephone 0171-351 7811

Marie Curie Cancer Care

Marie Curie Cancer Care, the UK's largest and most comprehensive cancer care charity, helps people with cancer by:

Offering with over 5,000 Marie Curie Nurses nationwide giving practical nursing care at home to people with cancer, without charge to the patient.

Providing specialised medical, nursing and paramedical care in 11 Marie Curie Hospice Centres throughout the UK.

Investigating the causes, prevention and detection of cancer through research at the Marie Curie Research Institute.

Improving the quality of cancer care through the education of health professionals.

For further information write to: **Marie Curie Cancer Care**, 28 Belgrave Square, London SW1X 8QG.

Telephone	0171-235-3325

Finally, a woman with breast cancer who has any queries about obtaining Social Security benefits should contact: **The National Association of Citizens Advice Bureaux**, 115–123 Pentonville Road, London N1 9LZ or look in their local telephone directory for details of their local Citizens Advice Bureau. There are 1500 bureaux nationwide and all of these can provide free, impartial, confidential advice and help.

10 Patient profiles

Name: ***Helen***

Age: ***46 years***

Occupation: ***Nurse***

Helen noticed a lump in her left breast.

On initial examination, it was considered that the lump was probably benign; however, a mammogram suggested a malignant tumour and this diagnosis was confirmed later by fine needle biopsy. As the tumour was small (less than 1.5cm), Helen was offered 'conservation' surgery and radiotherapy. The lump was removed and axillary lymph nodes sampled. No cancerous cells were detected in the lymph nodes and, as an oestrogen receptor test proved positive, Helen was offered adjuvant tamoxifen. As Helen was slightly anxious about the delay in her diagnosis, it was agreed that she should receive chemotherapy as well. She was given six outpatient-based treatments and did not experience any side-effects. Between the third and fourth cycles of chemotherapy, Helen received radiotherapy to the axilla and breast.

Helen's main complaint during chemotherapy was feeling slightly 'under the weather'.

Name:	***Sarah***
Age:	***51 years***
Occupation:	***Housewife***

Sarah went to her doctor when she noticed that her left breast was inflamed and swollen. She was sent to a breast cancer clinic where inoperable 'inflammatory' breast cancer was diagnosed by mammogram and clinical examination. A biopsy confirmed the presence of a hormone-insensitive tumour and, at the same time, a very fine tube was inserted into one of her veins to allow the continuous infusion of chemotherapy over the next 12 weeks. Sarah had to return to the breast cancer clinic on a weekly basis when she was given a second drug, her chemotherapy reservoir replenished and general health and disease response checked. After six weeks Sarah was experiencing fatigue and a sore mouth and had to wear a wig due to hair loss. However, she did not feel nauseous at any time and her tumour had shrunk dramatically. Twelve weeks after the original diagnosis, with a further week without therapy because of the recurrence of a sore mouth, the inflammation had disappeared and the tumour had shrunk sufficiently to allow a mastectomy to be performed. This surgery was followed by radiotherapy. Two years later Sarah remains well, is taking tamoxifen and has no evidence of active disease.

Name: ***Mabel***

Age: ***81 years***

Occupation: ***Unknown***

Mabel was referred to hospital with a 4cm mass in the left breast.

This mass was found to be malignant. Further staging tests showed no disease at other sites, but the breast mass was large and a mastectomy would have been necessary to control the disease in her breast. However, Mabel started to take tamoxifen by mouth and, after six weeks, the tumour was beginning to show a substantial reduction in size.

After a further six weeks, the tumour had shrunk sufficiently to allow a lumpectomy to be performed thus avoiding full removal of the breast by mastectomy.

The lumpectomy went smoothly and Mabel remains well two years later; she is still taking tamoxifen.

Name:	***Natalie***
Age:	***38 years***
Occupation:	***Housewife***

Natalie presented with a 2cm tumour of the right breast.

Following a needle biopsy and mammography, it was confirmed that Natalie had breast cancer. The cancer specialist did not consider that the cancer was extensive; however, it was not possible to perform a breast-conserving procedure due to the position of the tumour and Natalie had a mastectomy and axillary lymph node 'sampling'. The tumour proved to be hormone sensitive, with one axillary lymph node involved. In view of the extent of the disease and the hormone profile, it was recommended that Natalie should receive radiotherapy to the axilla and she was then offered ovariectomy to reduce the risk of recurrence.

Later, Natalie had a cosmetic breast reconstruction and her appearance and cosmetic result were very good. She remains well, but continues to experience some menopausal symptoms one year after surgery.

11 Answers to questions you may be asking yourself

I have a lump in my breast. I am frightened to tell anyone in case I have cancer. What shall I do?

No matter how you feel, you should see your family doctor as soon as you possibly can. The great majority of breast lumps are benign and not cancerous. Even if you do have breast cancer, the earlier you receive the right sort of treatment the more likely you are to make a full recovery. Do not delay in arranging to see your doctor.

If I have a mammogram regularly, will I be exposed to too much radiation?

Radiation exposure from modern mammogram equipment is minimal. It is far more dangerous *not* to find a breast cancer in its earliest stages than to be exposed to a low dose of radiation.

If I do not feel any lumps in my breasts, do I really need to have a mammogram?

A mammogram can detect a breast cancer as much as two years before it can be felt. Early detection of such a tumour gives a better chance of complete removal.

My mother died of breast cancer before she reached the age of 50 years. Am I likely to get breast cancer too?

It appears that a proportion of breast cancer cases is linked to factors that can be inherited by one generation from the previous one. Women with first-degree relatives who have had breast cancer at a relatively early age may themselves have a 50% risk of contracting the disease. Mothers are termed 'first-degree relative', as are sisters and daughters. So, while you are not necessarily going to get breast cancer, you do have a greater likelihood of doing so than the rest of the population. All women, but particularly those in your situation, should examine their breasts for lumps (in the week immediately following the menstrual period is the best time) and make sure they participate in mammography screening programmes. Speak to your family doctor about this. It is anticipated that most major centres will provide information on how you can get advice from cancer genetic clinics which are being developed in most major cities (see Section 3). Information on breast examination should be available from the practice nurse at your doctor's surgery, at well woman clinics or from the organisations mentioned in Section 9 of this book.

I have been diagnosed as having breast cancer. Will I get better?

Many women who have had breast cancer live a normal lifespan. Present treatments offer a good prognosis, but you may require several types of treatment to have the best chance of avoiding the disease recurring.

Will I have to have a mastectomy?

This depends on the size, position and type of your breast cancer as well as the size of your breast. Many patients do not require a total mastectomy and current medical practice is to conserve as much of the breast as possible. Sometimes, however, a better cosmetic result is obtained by mastectomy and reconstruction.

Does radiotherapy cause long-term damage and disfigurement?

No. It is exceptionally uncommon for a patient to experience unpleasant effects and damage from modern radiotherapy techniques.

Hormonal treatment for breast cancer has caused flushing and other menopausal symptoms. Would hormonal replacement therapy (HRT) be recommended to deal with these symptoms?

Many doctors normally advise against HRT as the hormones may, theoretically, stimulate re-growth of the cancer. There is argument about this, but many doctors feel that it is best to avoid HRT and use other ways, for example changing the type of hormone therapy, to minimise these symptoms.

Will chemotherapy side-effects ever go away?

Most side-effects are very short-lived, although it may not seem like that at the time. Nausea and vomiting are controlled completely or very successfully in most patients. Hair loss is by no means universal, although it usually means that a wig is needed for a few months beyond the chemotherapy period. Suppression of the function of the ovaries, by chemotherapy, may mean that your periods do disappear during treatment. Often they come back, but for women in their late 30s and 40s, the menopause may occur early.

12 Glossary

Adjuvant therapy

Additional or complementary treatment that is usually given after surgery. In terms of breast cancer, it may consist of chemotherapy, hormone therapy or radiotherapy.

Axillary lymph nodes

The lymph nodes (or lymph glands) in the underarm area.

Benign

A relatively harmless swelling or tumour that does not spread into the surrounding area or to other parts of the body. A benign tumour does not recur after surgical removal.

Biopsy

Removal of a small piece of tissue for examination by a pathologist.

Breast conservation

Removal of the tumour while retaining or conserving as much of the breast as possible.

CMF

A chemotherapy treatment using three drugs: cyclophosphamide, methotrexate and 5-fluorouracil

Computed tomography (CT)

A method of examining or scanning sites deep within the body.

Genetic disorder

An abnormality that arises in the genes in the nucleus of a cell. Genes determine an individual's characteristics, which are inherited from previous generations.

Hormone tests

Tests performed on tissue removed by biopsy to determine whether the presumed cancer is likely to be sensitive to hormone treatment.

Lumpectomy

Removal of a breast lump (rather than complete removal of the breast or mastectomy) as surgical treatment for breast cancer.

Lymph glands or lymph nodes

Part of the lymphatic system connected by minute lymph vessels. They are vitally concerned with fighting infection and disease in all areas of the body.

Lymphoedema

Swelling of the arm after surgery or radiotherapy for breast cancer. It occurs because the lymph is not draining adequately from the arm, due to damage to the underarm lymph nodes.

Magnetic resonance imaging (MRI)

A method of diagnosis that is useful for examining sites deep within the body. This imaging technique is performed in a 'scanner'.

Malignant

A tumour or swelling which is made up of abnormal cells that have the ability to spread into the surrounding tissues and to other parts of the body.

Mammography

An x-ray examination of the breast.

Mastectomy

Removal of the breast by surgery.

Metastases

Secondary tumours that develop when cancer cells invade blood vessels or lymph channels near the site of origin (the primary site) and are carried to other parts of the body.

Needle aspiration biopsy

Removal of material from a suspicious lump using a needle and syringe. A small amount of local anaesthetic may be used.

Neoplasm

A term that is often used interchangeably with cancer.

Oncologist

A doctor who specialises in the treatment of cancer.

Ovariectomy

Surgical removal of the ovaries. This is also termed oöphorectomy.

Pathological diagnosis

Examination of cells removed by biopsy to determine whether a tumour is benign or malignant.

Prognosis

The expert's opinion of the probable course and outcome of any illness, based on the relevant and attainable facts of each individual case.

Radiotherapy

Treatment using radiation, often given after surgery to help with eradication of any remaining cancer cells.

Secondary breast cancer

The spread of cancer cells from one body organ to another, not directly connected with it, is called metastasis and results in secondary cancers (or metastases).

Systemic treatment

Treatment of the whole body rather than local therapy to only the affected area.

Tumour

A tumour is a swelling caused by an abnormal cell multiplying to produce millions of cells that form a lump.

Ultrasound screening

A method being used more frequently for breast cancer diagnosis.

Zoladex® (Zeneca Pharma) is a registered trademark for goserelin.
Nolvadex® (Zeneca Pharma), **Emblon**® (Berk Pharmaceuticals Ltd) and **Oestrifen**® (Ashbourne Pharmaceuticals Ltd) are registered trademarks for tamoxifen.
Tamofen™ (Pharmacia Ltd) is a trademark for tamoxifen.
Provera®, **Depo-Provera**® (Upjohn Ltd) and **Farlutal**® (Pharmacia Ltd) are registered trademarks for medroxyprogesterone acetate.
Megace® (Bristol-Myers Squibb Pharmaceuticals) is a registered trademark for megestrol acetate.
Orimeten® (Ciba Pharmaceuticals) is a registered trademark for aminoglutethimide.
Lentaron® (Ciba Pharmaceuticals) is a registered trademark for formestane.
Arimedex® (Zeneca) is a registered trademark for anastrozole.
Endoxana® (ASTA Medica Ltd) is a registered trademark for cyclophosphamide.
Maxtrex® (Pharmacia Ltd) is a registered trademark for methotrexate.
Fluoro-Uracil Roche® (Roche Products Limited) is a registered trademark for 5-fluorouracil.
Novantrone® (Lederle Laboratories) is a registered trademark for mitozantrone.
Pharmorubicin® (Pharmacia Ltd) is a registered trademark for epirubicin.
Oncovin® (Lilly Eli & Co. Ltd) is a registered trademark for vincristine.
Taxol™ (Bristol-Myers Squibb Pharmaceuticals Ltd) is a registered trademark for paclitaxel.
Taxotere® (Rhone-Poulenc Rorer Ltd) is a registered trademark for docetaxel.
Zavedos® (Pharmacia Ltd) is a registered trademark for idarubicin.

Index

Index *continued*